CONTENTS

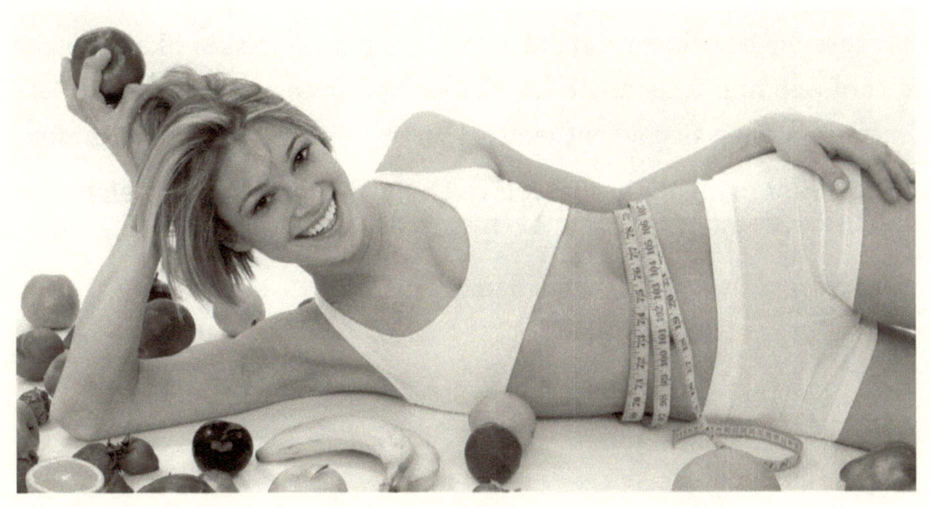

WEIGHT LOSS
DIET AND TIPS

Are you among those who are trying hard to lose weight even after following the diet and tips given by a dietician? Well, you are making some inconsiderable mistakes.

Here in this book, I will guide you about these mistakes which you have never thought can be the culprit in a way to weight loss.

These mistakes which I am highlighting are researched personally among 5 groups of 4 people each consisting of all age groups, adults from 18 to 50 years of age.

Under the guidance of a dietician, a variety of diet chart is prepared considering age and BMI, followed for 3 months, still weight loss is not observed in 2 groups while in the remaining 3 groups, drastic consistent change is visible after 2 months of dedication.

Why?

Because we have incorporated some negligible mistakes like the same diet of weight loss for all, the same food options no variety, same or less exercise, and no alcohol botheration, in the routine of the first 2 groups.

Here I want to highlight that it is not only diet that leads to weight loss but there are many other factors responsible too.

Let's discuss these mistakes in detail.

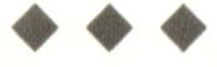

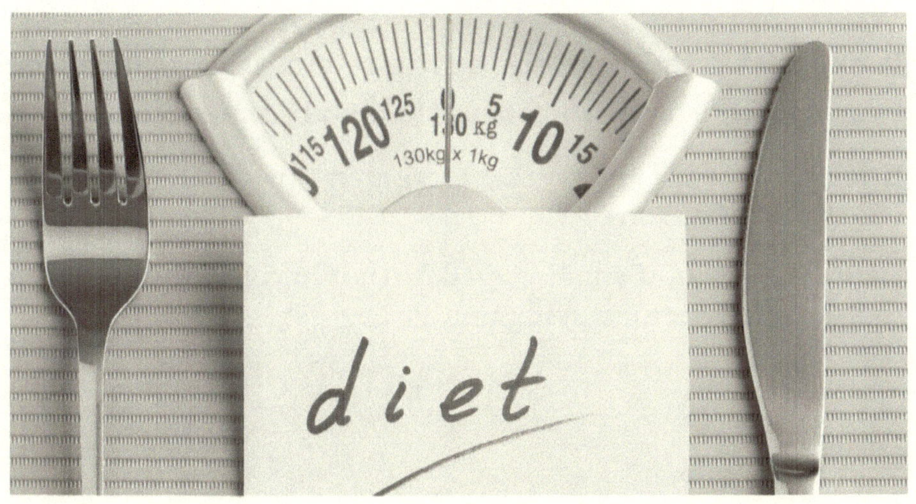

13 SURPRISING REASONS WHY YOUR DIET IS NOT WORKING

There are many types of diets approved by dieticians to stay healthy and maintain normal body weight.

But, let me tell you that there is no such diet that works for all. As everyone is different, there is no such diet that suits all.

Whether you are on Atkins, paleo, or keto, and if it is not working for you then there might be some surprising reasons behind it.

Keep in mind that no diet will let you drastically lose weight in a matter of weeks.

According to the Council on Size & Weight Discrimination, within one to five years 95% of dieters regain their lost weight regardless of the diet or exercises that they follow.

It means that the same diet and same exercising routine stop working after a few years because the body becomes habitual.

If you are on a diet and see that there aren't any results it could be due to a lot of reasons.

Here are a few of them discussed furthur in coming chapters, so that you can figure out systematically.

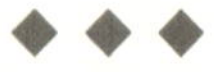

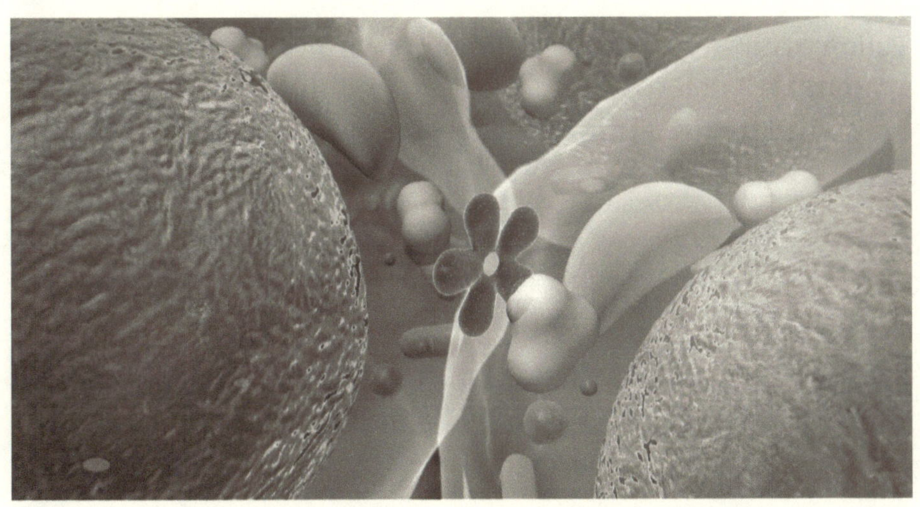

GENETICS AND HORMONES REGULATE BODY WEIGHT

Studies reveal that everyone has their own body weight which is regulated by genes and hormones at some point.

You can understand this by the example of rubber if the rubber is stretched the greater the resistance and it will again come back to its original shape similarly when we control weight through food and exercise then we are stretching the body out of our comfort zone then greater the desire to come back.

This theory proves that the greater we work hard the greater body tries to come back to natural.

Then what should one do?

Follow intuitive eating, eat for physical rather than emotional reasons.

- Intuitive eating: Eat only when you feel hungry and eat as much you want and what you want. But stop when you are full.
- Emotion goes for unhealthy and tasty foods but eats for physical reasons which mean eating nourishing food that is required by your body.

This does not mean stopping yourself from desserts or fries but sometimes you can have it in moderation.

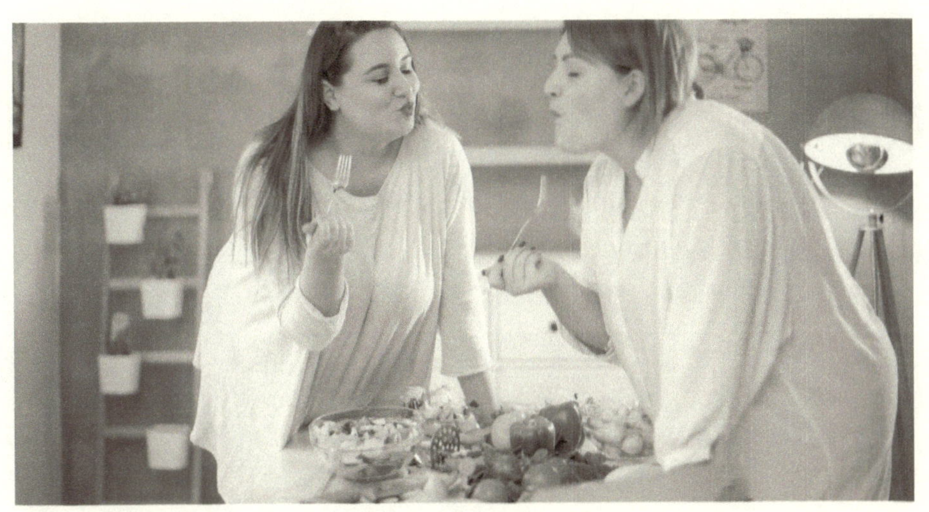

EAT FOOD YOU ENJOY WITHOUT GUILT

N ow, it is clear that diets are not linked with long-term weight loss.

This strategy of dieting, and restricting yourself from food will worsen your weight problem.

Though you may see the benefits, in long run this will also fade away as the body will become habitual of the diet you are following and weight will again start increasing.

The solution is eating everything but in moderation and with limitations.

Do not force restriction too hard just be aware of quantity .

Make yourself aware of of the healthy variations.

Incorporate everything in your diet in moderation and enjoy it without guilt or overthinking.

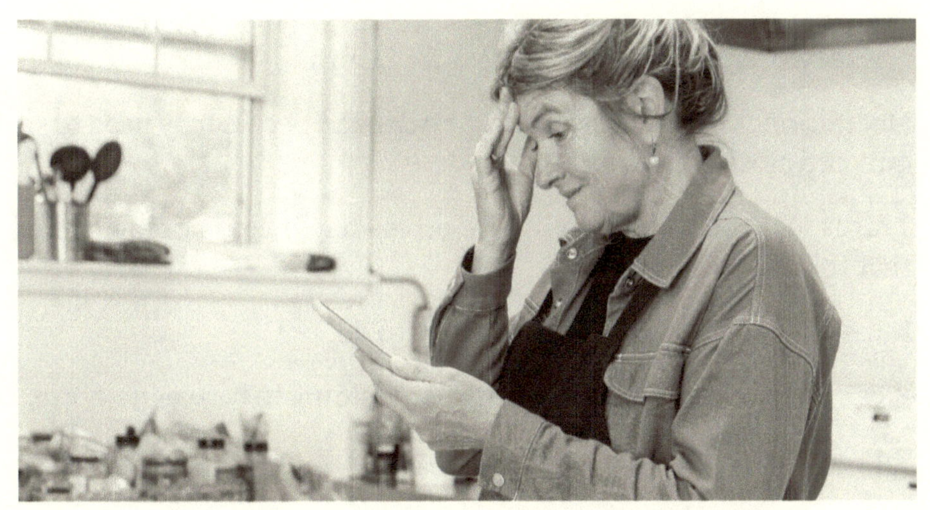

KEEP YOUR STRESS
UNDER CONTROL

Keep your stress hormone i.e. cortisol under check. When there is a lot of stress then it triggers cortisol secretion.

The elevated levels of cortisol affect the metabolism and appetite increases.

Research also reveals that chronic stress pumped the rate at which new fat cells are formed.

Straight forward to get more stress more chances of fat increase.

In todays life its very hard to avoid stress.

Stressful situation comes and goes but what you need to learn is the stress management.

Find time for yourself be it for 15 minutes.

Meditate and Exercise.

These two things are the wonders for health.

Meditation is for relaxing mind, you doesn't necessarily need to sit quit and close your eyes.

This is just the way to do it. The other may include doing things that relaxes your mind.

It means your hobby, which you love to do.

It can be listening songs, painting, or residing in between nature.

This will surely keep stress under control.

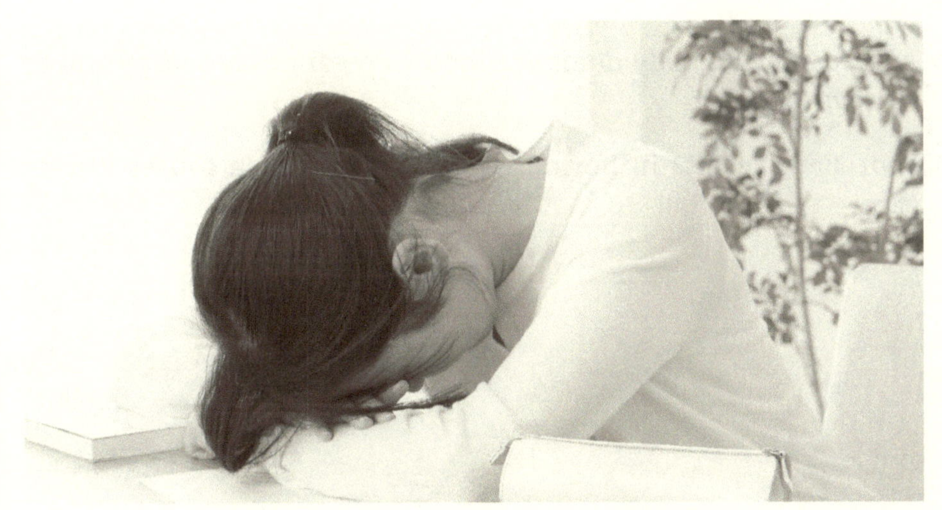

LACK OF SLEEP

Sleep deprivation disturbs the hunger hormones (ghrelin) which lead to increased appetite.

This will lead to hormonal imbalance and weight gain. Get enough sleep to maintain weight.

The University of Chicago found that when people are sleep-deprived then they eat 600 calories more than usual.

So, the fat cells increase. Also, the Leptin hormone's secretion is hampered (which decreases your appetite).

As a result, weight loss progress will be hindered and soon you will be on the path of obesity.

In simple words, the less you sleep the more you eat.

The body will demand more food to compensate less sleep.

Actually when you do not get proper sleep then you feel lethargic, less energetic, and drowned.

As a result, the body demands food to regain that energy and to remove lethargy.

Poor sleep results in hormonal disbalance which causes weight gain.

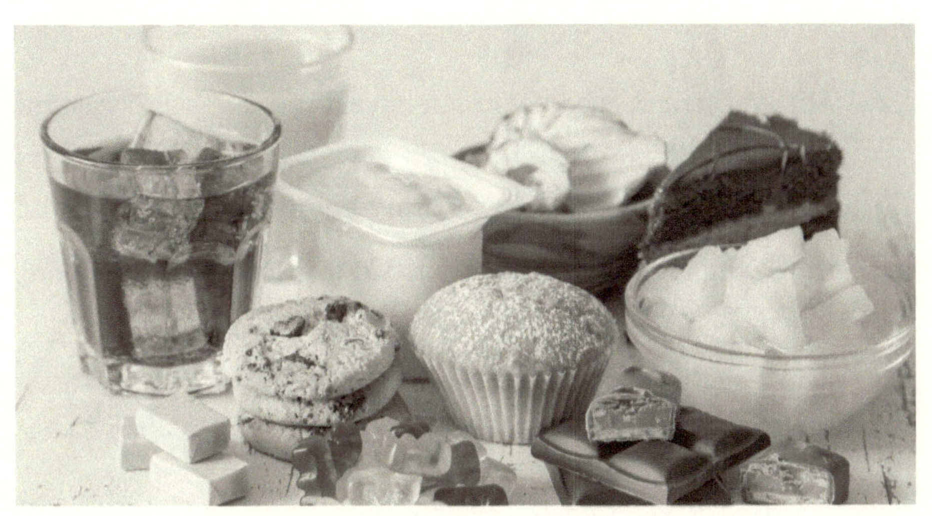

EATING TOO MUCH SUGAR AND PROCESSED FOOD

Never stop yourself from eating anything until you have major diseases like diabetes or heart problem.

But always remember not to indulge in oily, processed, salt, and sugar-based products as they cause high blood pressure, cholesterol, and many other diseases.

Control your salt intake as well if you want to maintain your weight. Too much sodium is also not good for bones and the heart as well.

Eating too much of them will affect your weight and also your health.

Processed food has harmful preservatives and chemicals which should be avoided for being healthy.

Excess of everything is bad. You can have it in parties or occasions but only sometimes.

Do not make it a habit and neither crave yourself for indulging it.

Remember sugar and processed food do no good to your body except satisfying the tongue.

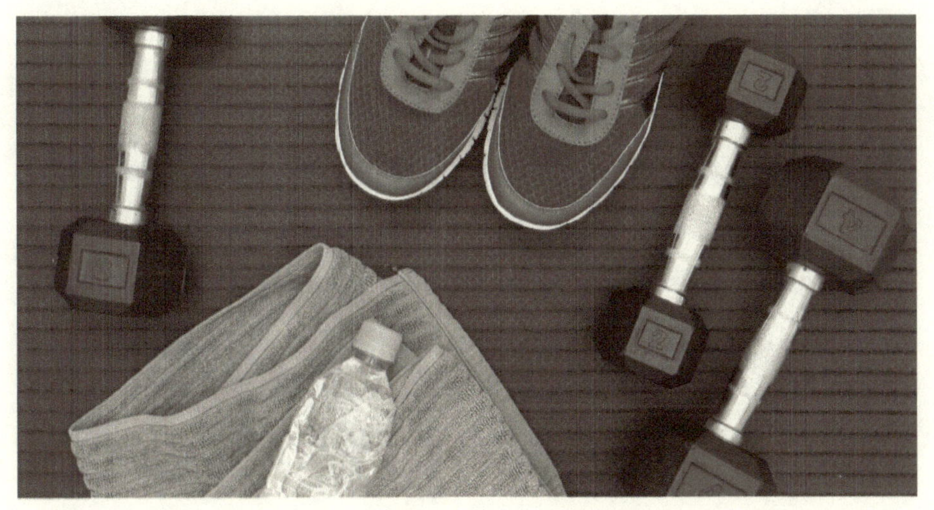

LACK OF EXERCISE
IN ROUTINE

It is very important to burn the calories, the stubborn fat that you consumed.

Exercise is a must even if you are eating healthy. This will help you maintain proper weight and health.

If your main purpose of exercising is weight loss then do not forget to lift weights. Strength training is an actual way to lose fat.

According to the mayo clinic leaving exercise is the surprising reason behind weight regain.

Also, try to do cardio. Studies say that it helps to reduce fat around the midsection.

Remeber movement is very essential for body. Even a troll for 15minutes add health benefits.

For weight loss running, swimming, dancing and all the other forms of cardio like climbing stairs etc results good.

Weight training also helps in much faster fat loss.

The only thing is consistency that brings the result. Along with consistency do not forget to add a recovery day to your schedule.

You might be thinking about recovery day now? Well just take a day off from exercises too.

Basically you can call it a rest day. It gives body chance to recover and relaxes muscles too. It help in avoiding sprain and muscle rupture.

Never miss to warm up and stretch body before starting any form of exercise.

And in the same way relax and cool down body after performing exercises.

For better results and guidance exercises should be done under the guidance of a trainer .

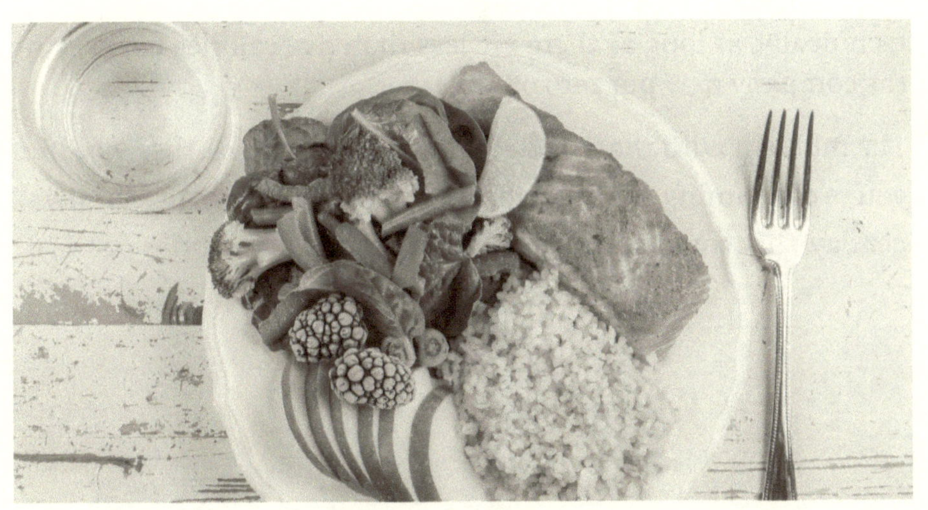

CHECK YOUR PORTION

Eating too much or too less will affect health, even if you are opting for healthy foods like nuts, fruits, seeds, and guacamole.

Consume fats, also carbohydrates, but in required amounts. Research reveals that when you avoid fats than it triggers you to eat more and you binge on junk food instead of a bowl full of veggies.

Bad fats should be avoided and good fats should be incorporated into a diet like avocados, eggs, and nuts.

Checking the portion size of food is essential but if you are relying on sugar-free foods you think you saved calories?

Well, that's not the case. They also use sugar alcohols, which contain one to three calories per gram compared to carbohydrates which provide four calories per gram.

The serving sizes often list zero calories/grams of sugar because, technically, as long as there are less than five calories per serving the company may put zero on the label.

The problem with that? The serving size is tiny! In other words, if you're consuming sugar alcohol in multiple servings per meal and per day, that could quickly lead to an extra 100+ calories per day!

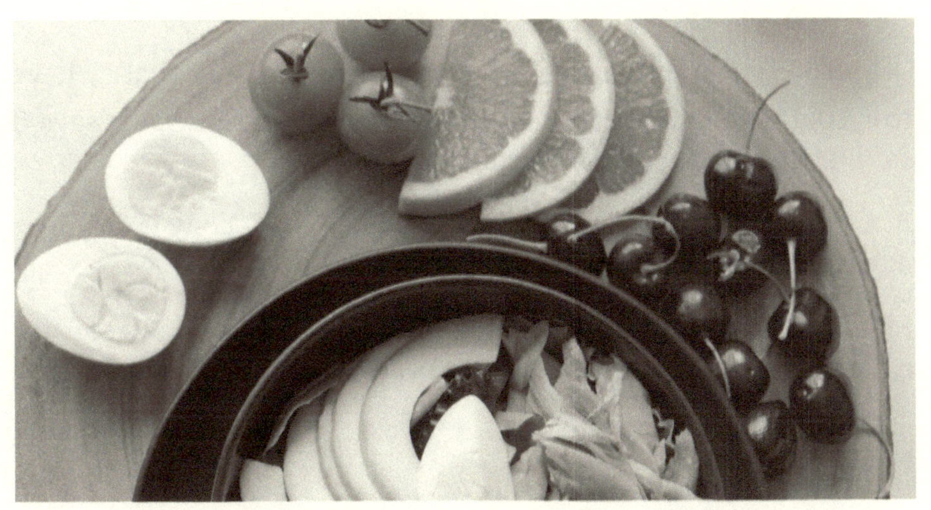

VARIETY IS KEY

Do not be on a specific diet for too long as it's all about making lifestyle changes. Gradually for more sustainable results than just juggling at different times.

Everybody is unique and their nutrition requirements differ.

If you follow the same diet for long then it will stop giving you the result.

Make changes to your diet keeping in mind the calorie intake and calorie burnt.

Without consulting a dietician avoid making changes to your food.

Dietician and health experts can guide you about the needs of your body judging your BMI.

Body is your only place to live and you have to take care of it always.

We usually get influenced when somebody tell us that "I have lost 10kg's weight following keto diet" or when somebody says "I found myself better with vegan diet."

But my advice is that never follow anyone. Every body is different and its requirement is different too.

Please do not experiment on your body with diets. Always consult a doctor before following any type of diet.

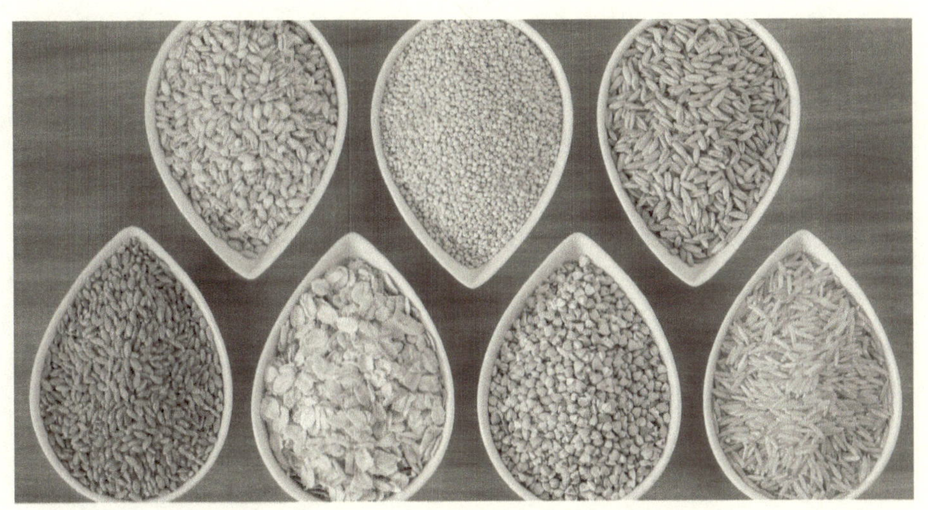

EAT SUFFICIENT PROTEIN AND WHOLE GRAIN

Low protein intake can be one reason for weight gain. Rich protein diets like Fish and whole grains must be included in the diet to maintain proper weight.

According to National Institute of Health observational studies suggest that higher whole grain intake is associated with lower risk of weight gain.

As per studies the sufficient quantity of protein that an average man should take daily is 56gm and for average woman is 46gm.

Protein has a high satiety effect, meaning it can help you feel full and satisfied for longer periods of time.

This can help reduce overall calorie intake, which is essential for weight management.

Additionally, protein can help preserve muscle mass during weight loss, which can help maintain a healthy metabolism.

Whole grains also have a high satiety effect, thanks to their high fiber content.

Fiber is an indigestible carbohydrate that adds bulk to food, making you feel full and satisfied.

Whole grains also tend to be lower in calories than refined grains, which can help with weight management.

Also, whole grains have a lower glycemic index than refined grains, which means they are digested and absorbed more slowly.

This can help regulate blood sugar levels and prevent spikes in insulin, which can contribute to weight gain.

Furthermore, a diet that is rich in protein and whole grains can help improve overall nutrient intake and support a healthy metabolism, which can further contribute to weight management.

Hence, consuming sufficient protein and whole grains can be an effective strategy for maintaining a healthy weight and reducing the risk of weight gain over time.

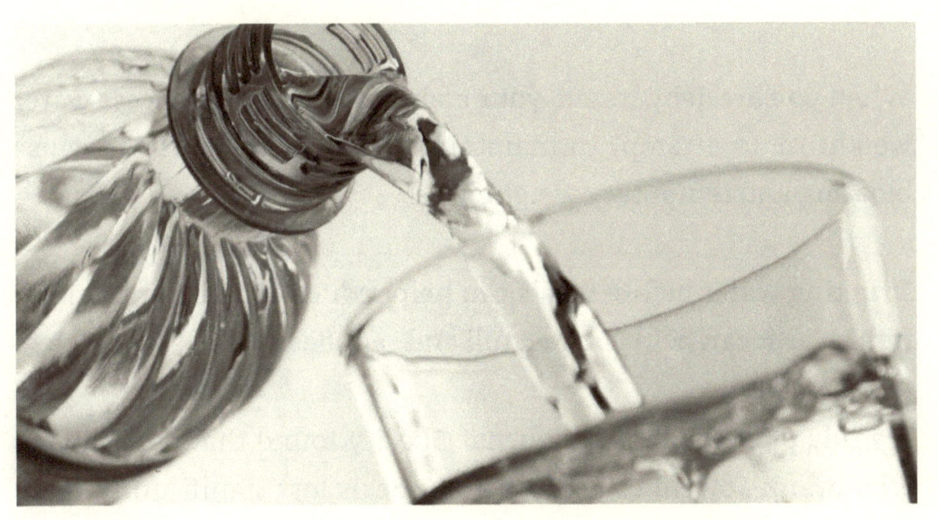

NOT DRINKING
ENOUGH WATER

This is surprisingly true. To avoid excessive eating it is advised to drink a glass of water before meals. This will reduce your calorie intake.

It will also increase the number of calories you burn. So, drink before you feel thirsty.

Not drinking enough water can be related to weight gain.

This is because water plays an important role in several bodily functions, including metabolism, digestion, and the elimination of waste.

When you are dehydrated, your body may slow down its metabolic rate in an effort to conserve water. This can make it more difficult to burn calories and lose weight.

When you are dehydrated, your body may hold on to excess water weight in an attempt to maintain fluid balance. This can cause bloating and temporary weight gain.

Drinking water before meals can help reduce appetite and calorie intake, as it can help you feel full and satisfied.

A study published in the journal Obesity found that participants who drank 500 ml of water before meals lost significantly more weight than those who did not.

It is important to note that drinking water alone is not a magic solution for weight loss.

However, staying hydrated and consuming adequate amounts of water throughout the day can support overall health and help facilitate weight management.

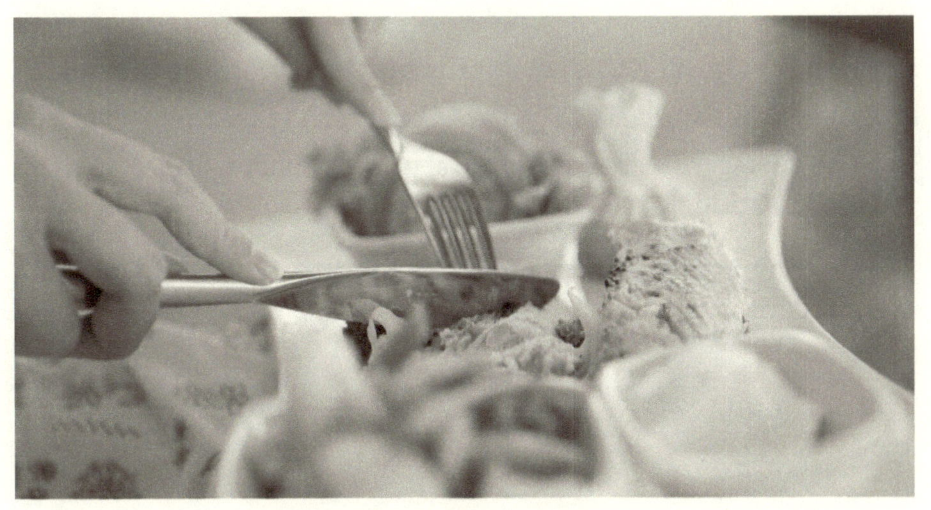

NOT EATING
MINDFULLY

You must have heard to eat in a relaxed mood and we usually eat freely with our family and friends or at parties.

There is nothing bad in it. The only point to consider is mindful eating.

What is that?

Mindful eating is alert eating. Eat with zero distractions.

For example, eating while watching a movie, or your favorite show on tv makes you eat more because your mind is not aware it is distracted.

As a result, no signal is sent to the brain that your stomach is full and it results in overeating.

Eat slowly and chew thoroughly. This will make you feel full faster.

This is very true and is scientifically proven (according to research highlighted in studies of Harvard University) that the slower you eat the faster you feel full and also proper chewing results in better digestion.

Stop eating when you feel full. This will surely save you from weight gain.

Practice mindful eating because it can help prevent weight gain by:

* Encouraging you to pay attention to hunger and fullness cues, which can help prevent overeating.

* Promoting awareness of the food you eat and how it affects your body, which can help you make healthier choices.

* Reducing stress-related eating by promoting a more relaxed and mindful approach to food.

* Encouraging you to savor and enjoy your food, which can lead to greater satisfaction and reduce the urge to overeat.

One important message to give about mindful eating is that it is not a diet, but rather a way of approaching food with greater awareness and attention.

Mindful eating is not about counting calories or restricting certain foods, but rather about tuning into your body's needs and preferences.

Another important message is that mindful eating can be

practiced in many different ways, such as by slowing down while eating, savoring the flavors and textures of food, and paying attention to hunger and fullness cues.

It is also important to note that practicing mindful eating may take time and patience, and it may require breaking old habits and patterns around food.

However, with practice, mindful eating can become a natural and enjoyable way of approaching food and can support overall health and wellbeing.

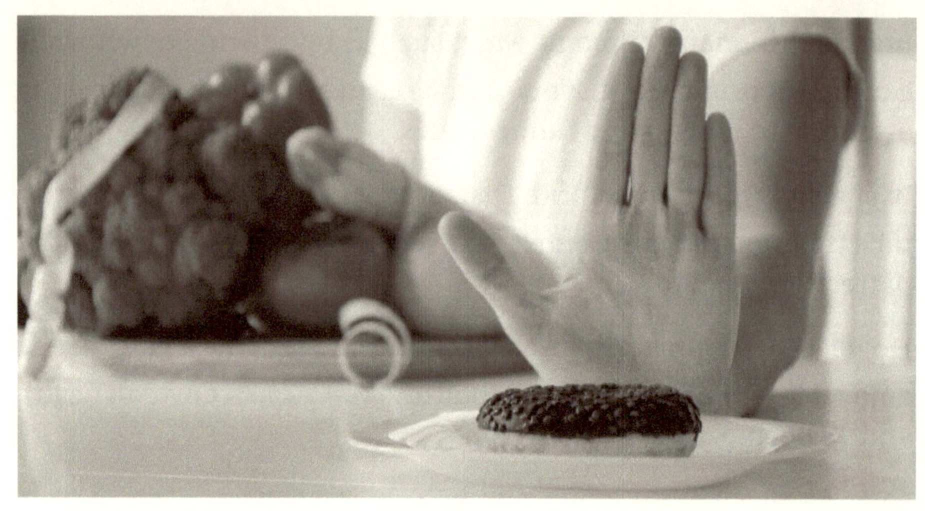

AVOID RESTRICTIVE DIETING

R estrictive dieting in the start will result in weight loss and you perceive the efforts as successful.

But you crave foods that are restricted.

When the gates to restricted foods are open we indulge without thinking and during this break you are likely to gain more weight.

Weight loss and then weight gain is a vicious cycle.

And again you go for restrictive dieting and in this way it becomes a vicious cycle.

Instead, it is advisable to go on dieting which controls your portion size.

There are several reasons why one should avoid restrictive dieting:

It can lead to nutrient deficiencies: Restrictive diets often eliminate entire food groups, which can lead to nutrient deficiencies if these nutrients are not obtained from other sources.

It can slow down metabolism: When you restrict your calorie intake too much, your body may slow down its metabolic rate in order to conserve energy. This can make it more difficult to lose weight and maintain weight loss over time.

It can lead to binge eating: Restrictive diets can create feelings of deprivation and lead to binge eating episodes, which can further contribute to weight gain.

It can negatively impact mental health: Restrictive dieting can create a preoccupation with food, as well as feelings of guilt and shame around eating. This can lead to poor body image and negatively impact mental health.

It is often unsustainable: Restrictive diets are often difficult to maintain over the long-term, which can lead to weight regain and a cycle of yo-yo dieting.

It is important to approach food and nutrition in a balanced and sustainable way, rather than through strict and rigid rules.

A flexible and mindful approach to eating can support overall health and wellbeing, while avoiding the negative consequences of restrictive dieting.

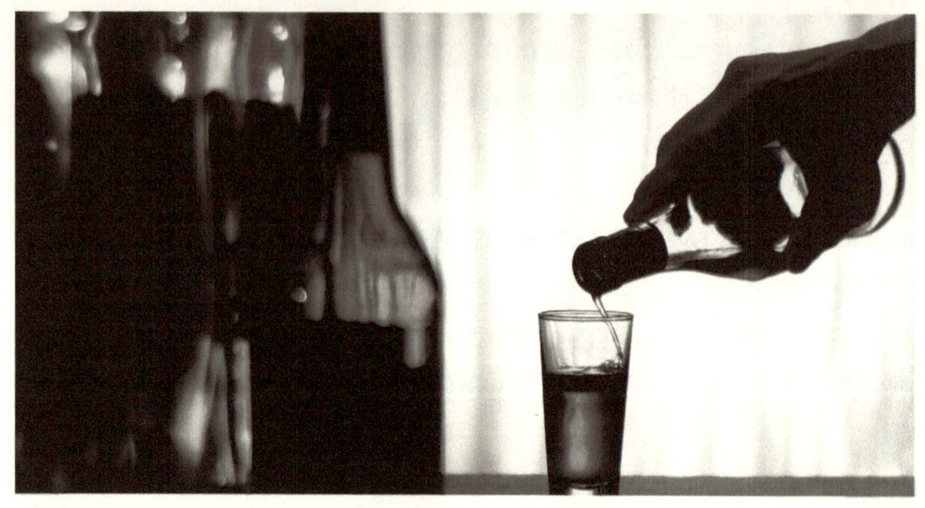

EXCESSIVE ALCOHOL

Drinking excessive alcohol is one of the reasons for weight gain.

It is high in calories.

The alcohol has about 7 calories per gram. Avoid it if you can for weight loss.

Excessive alcohol consumption can lead to weight gain.

This is because alcohol is high in calories, with 7 calories per gram, which is almost as much as fat, which has 9 calories per gram.

Consuming excessive amounts of alcohol can therefore contribute to a significant calorie intake, which can lead to weight gain over time.

Alcohol can stimulate the appetite and lead to overeating, as it can reduce inhibitions and increase the desire for high-calorie foods. This can further contribute to weight gain.

Alcohol can negatively affect metabolism, as the body prioritizes metabolizing alcohol over other nutrients. This can slow down the metabolism of carbohydrates and fats, which can contribute to weight gain.

In addition, some alcoholic beverages, such as beer and sweet mixed drinks, can be high in carbohydrates and sugars, which can also contribute to weight gain.

While moderate alcohol consumption may not lead to significant weight gain, excessive and regular consumption of alcohol can contribute to weight gain and other negative health consequences.

CONCLUSION

Weight loss is not an easy task and many of our daily habits and lifestyle routine can bring it to halt.

In an easy way, you can understand it as when your calorie intake is higher than the calorie burnt then weight gain occurs.

Try approaches such as mindful eating, eating more protein, and doing strength exercises.

So, all the above are outer excessive ways to control weight.

It's better to avoid them instead of being too late for them!

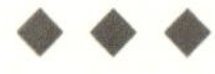